To parents and caregivers who help children overcome their fears.

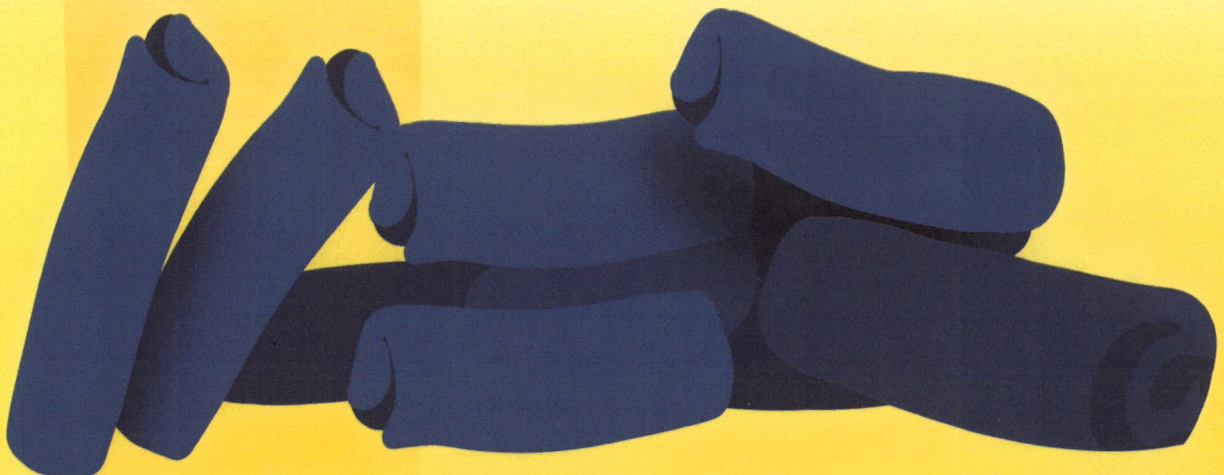

The main character of this book is based on the real-life personality of Samia Ali from Samia's Life

For information contact:
Samia's Life at www.samiaslife.com

Written and designed by Dr. Cymanthia Connell and Adam Ali
ISBN: Hardcopy   978-1-7346872-3-1
         Paperback 978-1-7346872-4-8
         Ebook   978-1-7346872-5-5

Library of Congress Control Number: 2020908642

Published by Cymanthia Connell, M.D., LLC
Atlanta, Georgia USA

Second Edition: June 2020

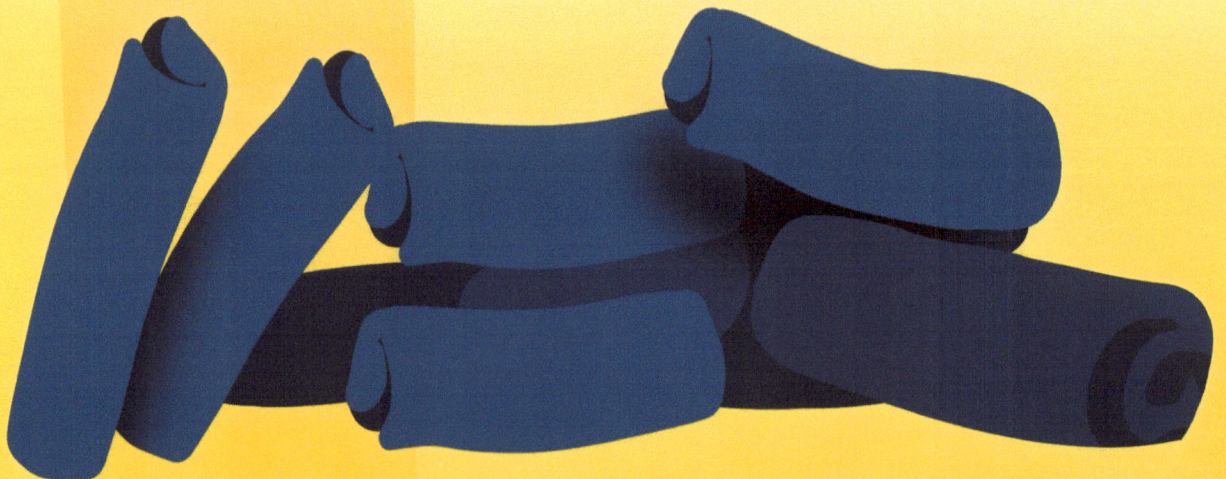

Samia's First Day at Gymnastics

By Dr. Cymanthia Connell
and Adam Ali

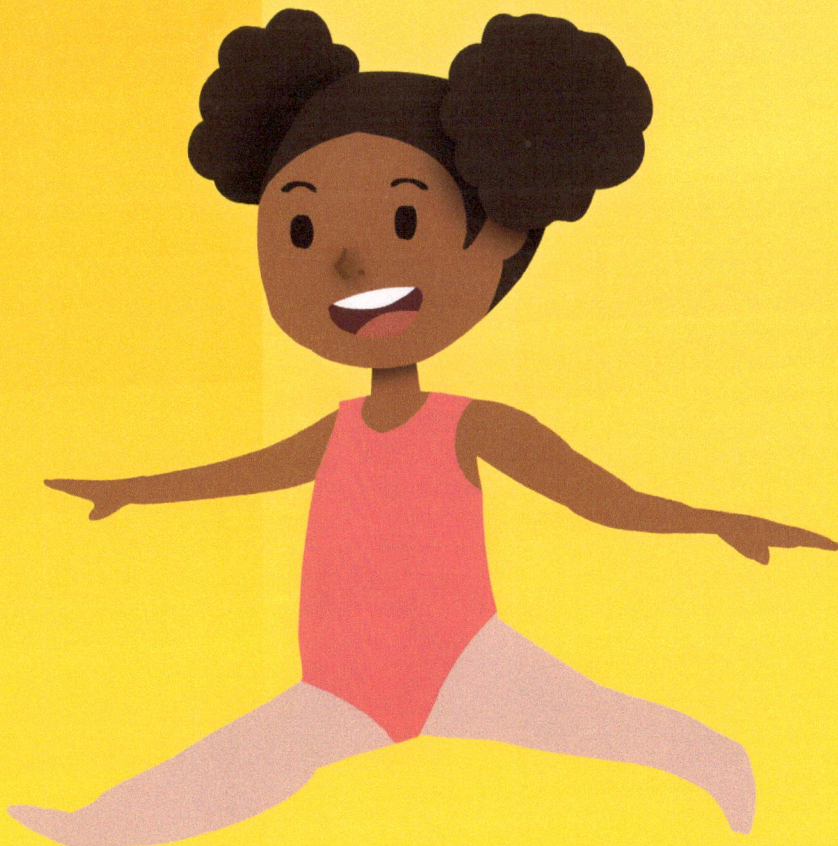

All summer long, Samia could not wait to start gymnastics class. She loved to do cartwheels and twirls!

"I cannot wait to show my new gymnastics coach my handstand," said Samia.

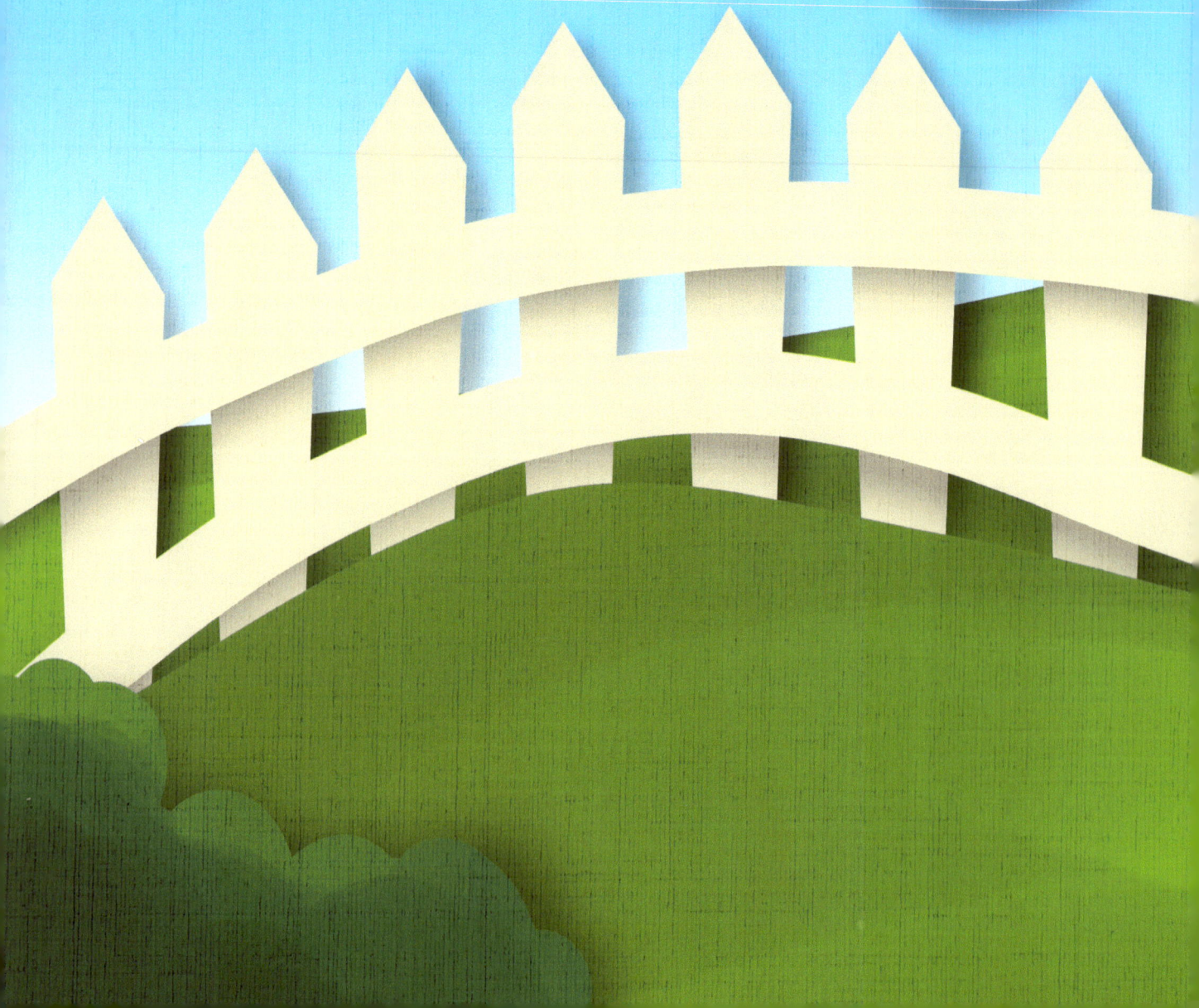

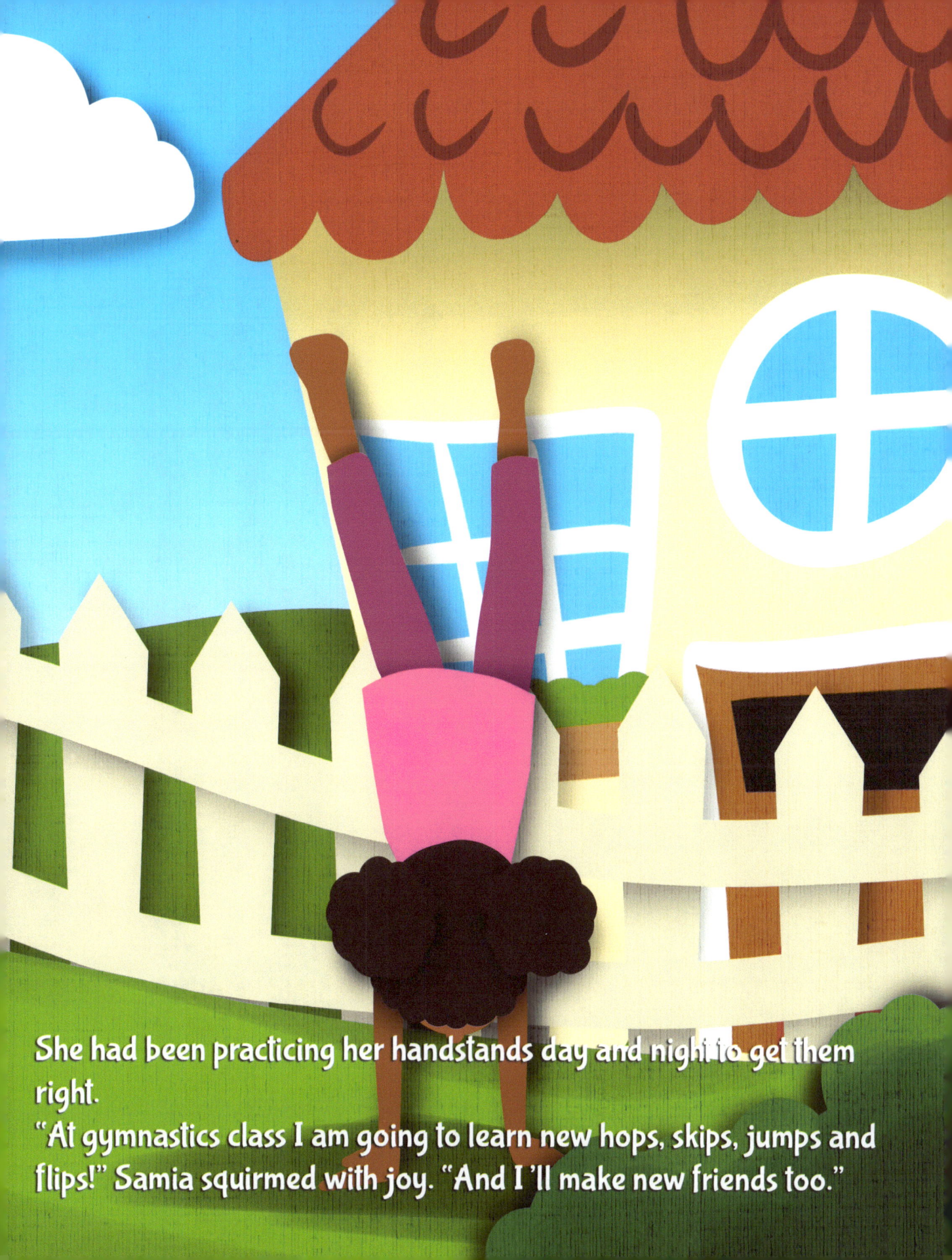

She had been practicing her handstands day and night to get them right.
"At gymnastics class I am going to learn new hops, skips, jumps and flips!" Samia squirmed with joy. "And I'll make new friends too."

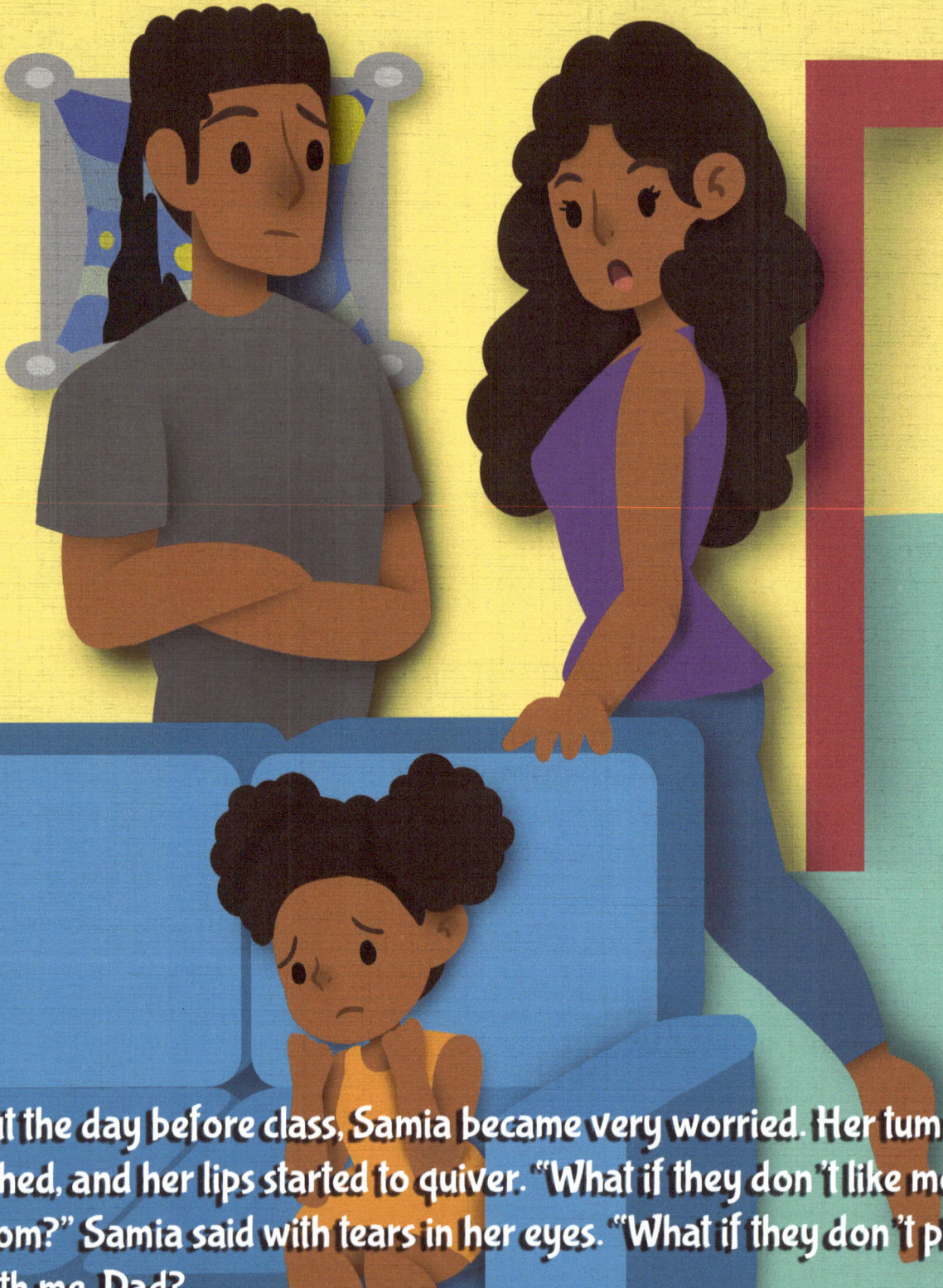

But the day before class, Samia became very worried. Her tummy ached, and her lips started to quiver. "What if they don't like me, Mom?" Samia said with tears in her eyes. "What if they don't play with me, Dad?

Samia's tears began to fall.

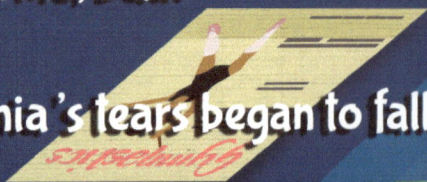

"I don't want to go" Samia whimpered. Samia's whimper became a cry. Samia's crying became a sob. She looked very uncomfortable. "But...but...but I don't want to go!" said Samia.

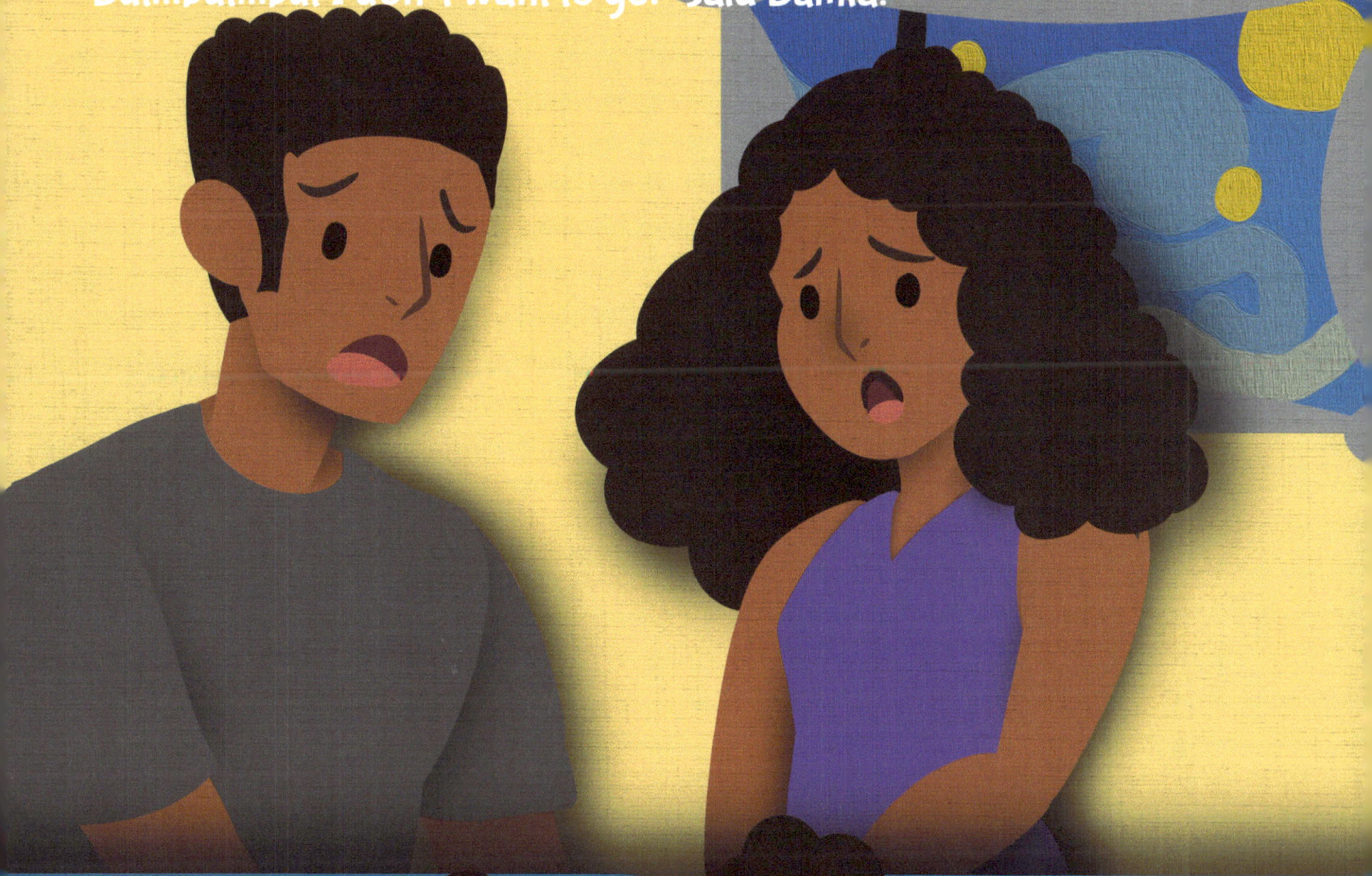

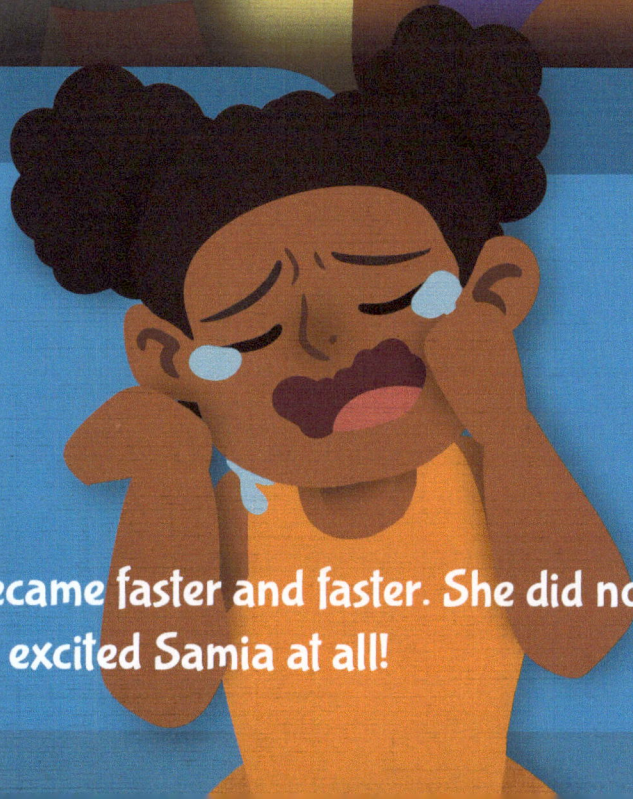

Her breathing became faster and faster. She did not look like the usual happy and excited Samia at all!

"I think today's the day we teach Samia deep breathing so that she can feel better," Dad said to Mom.

"Yes!" said Mom. "Let's play a game"

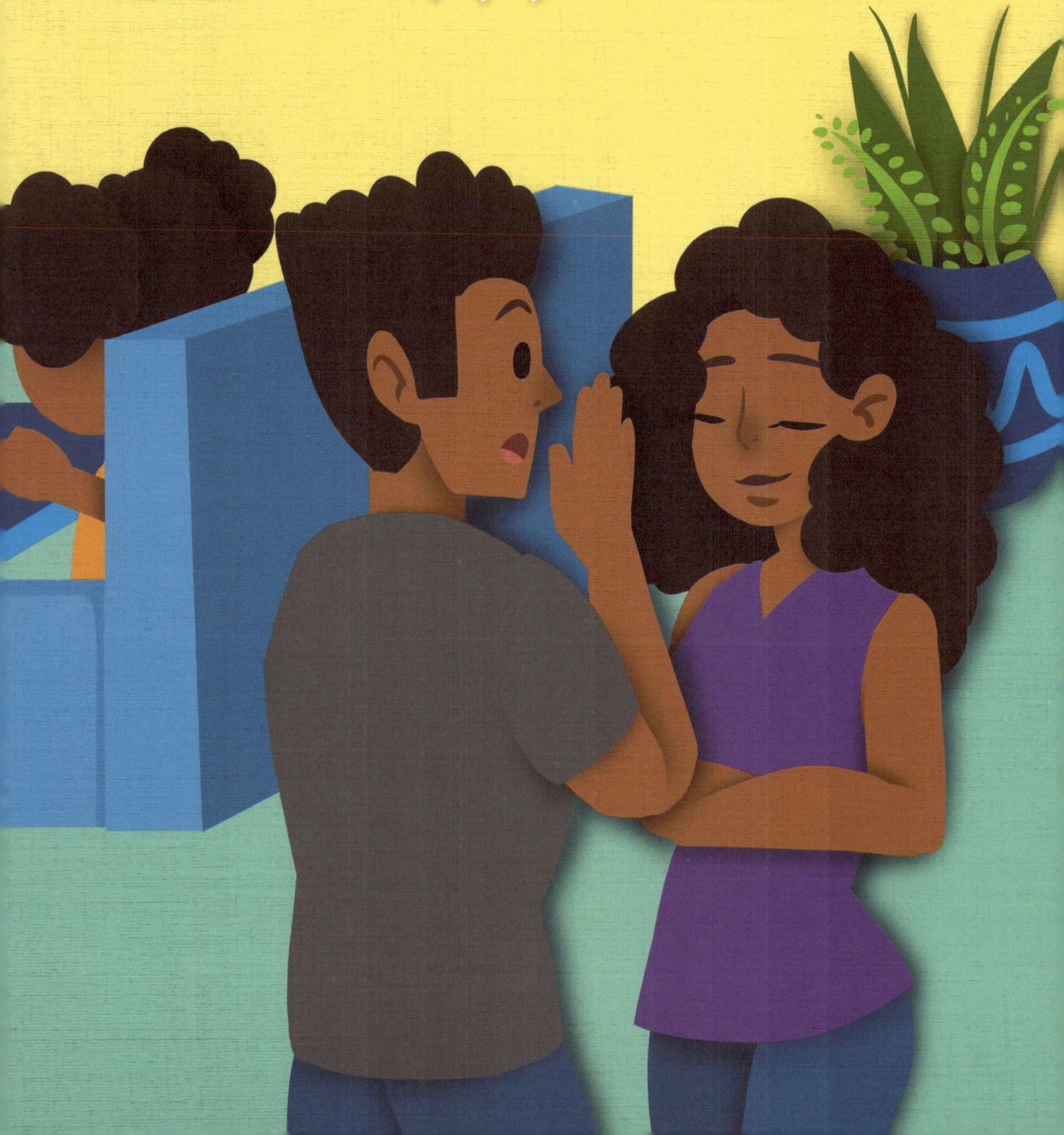

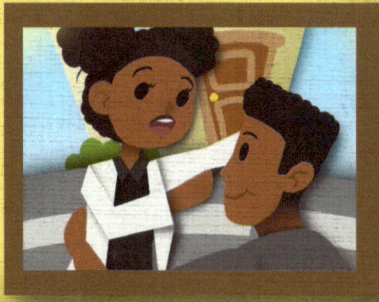

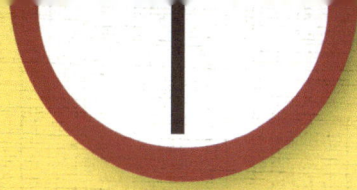

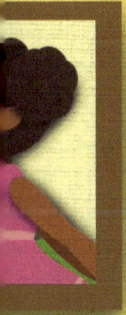

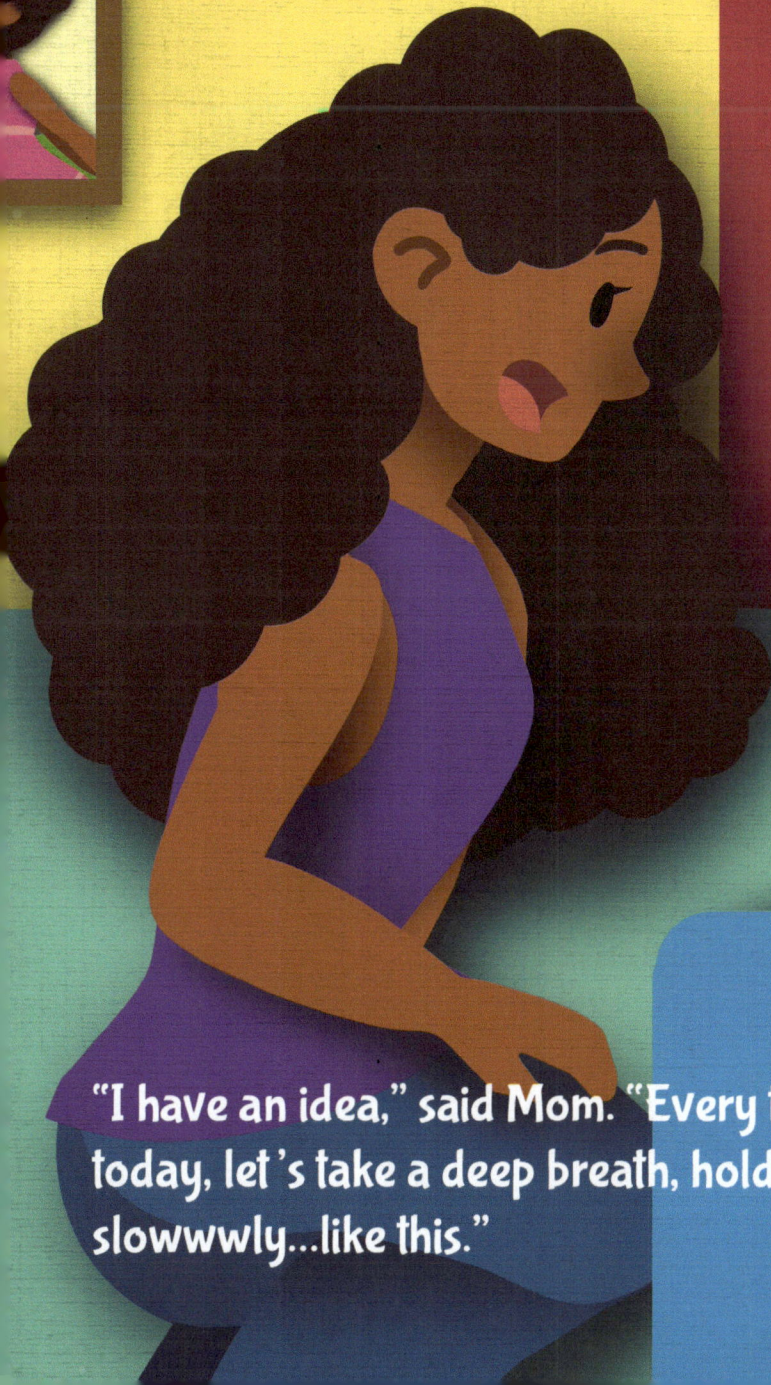

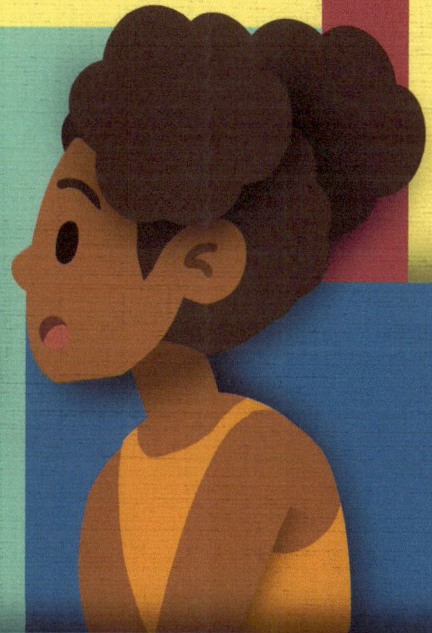

"I have an idea," said Mom. "Every time you feel a little nervous today, let's take a deep breath, hold it...and let it out slowwwly...like this."

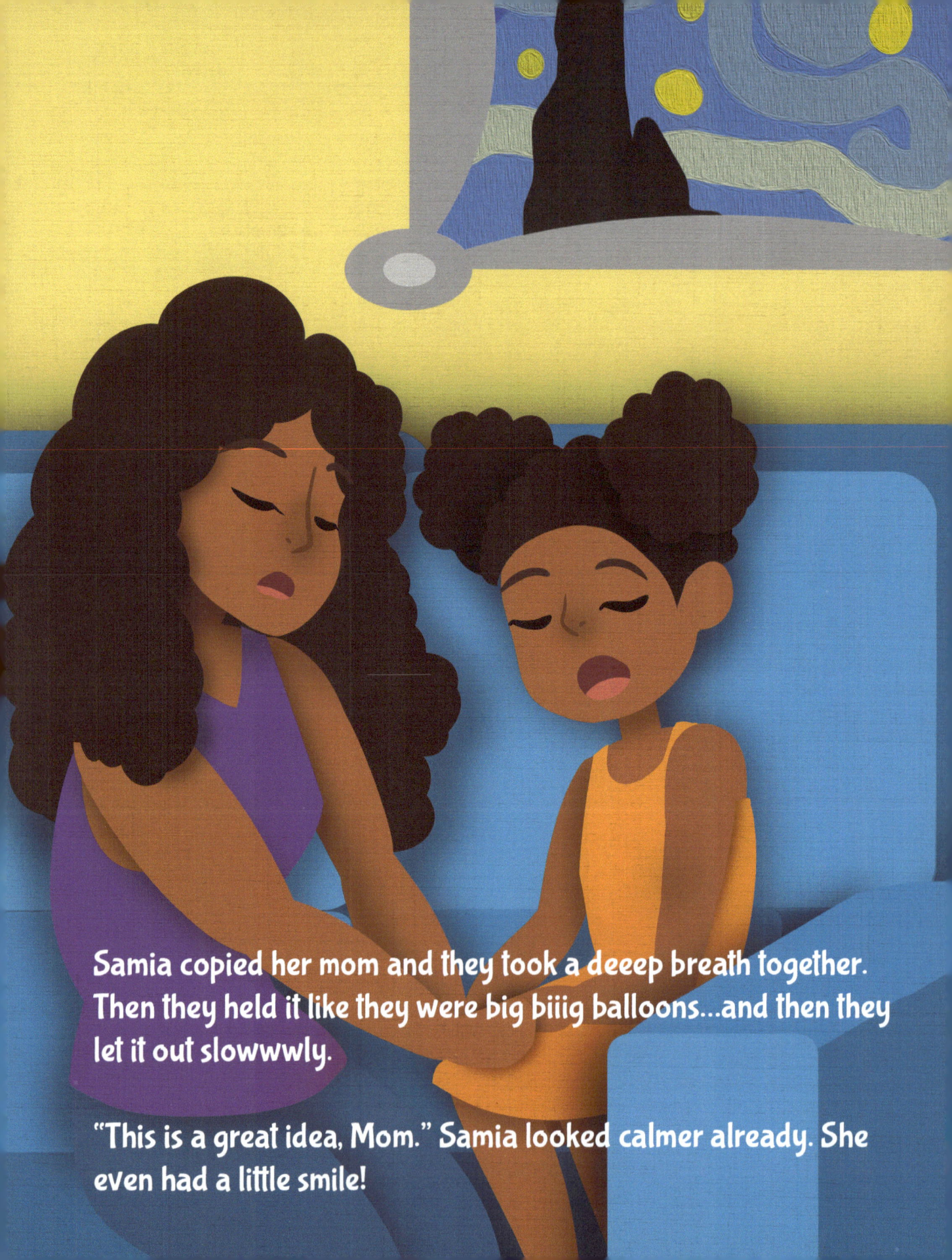

Samia copied her mom and they took a deeep breath together. Then they held it like they were big biiig balloons...and then they let it out slowwwly.

"This is a great idea, Mom." Samia looked calmer already. She even had a little smile!

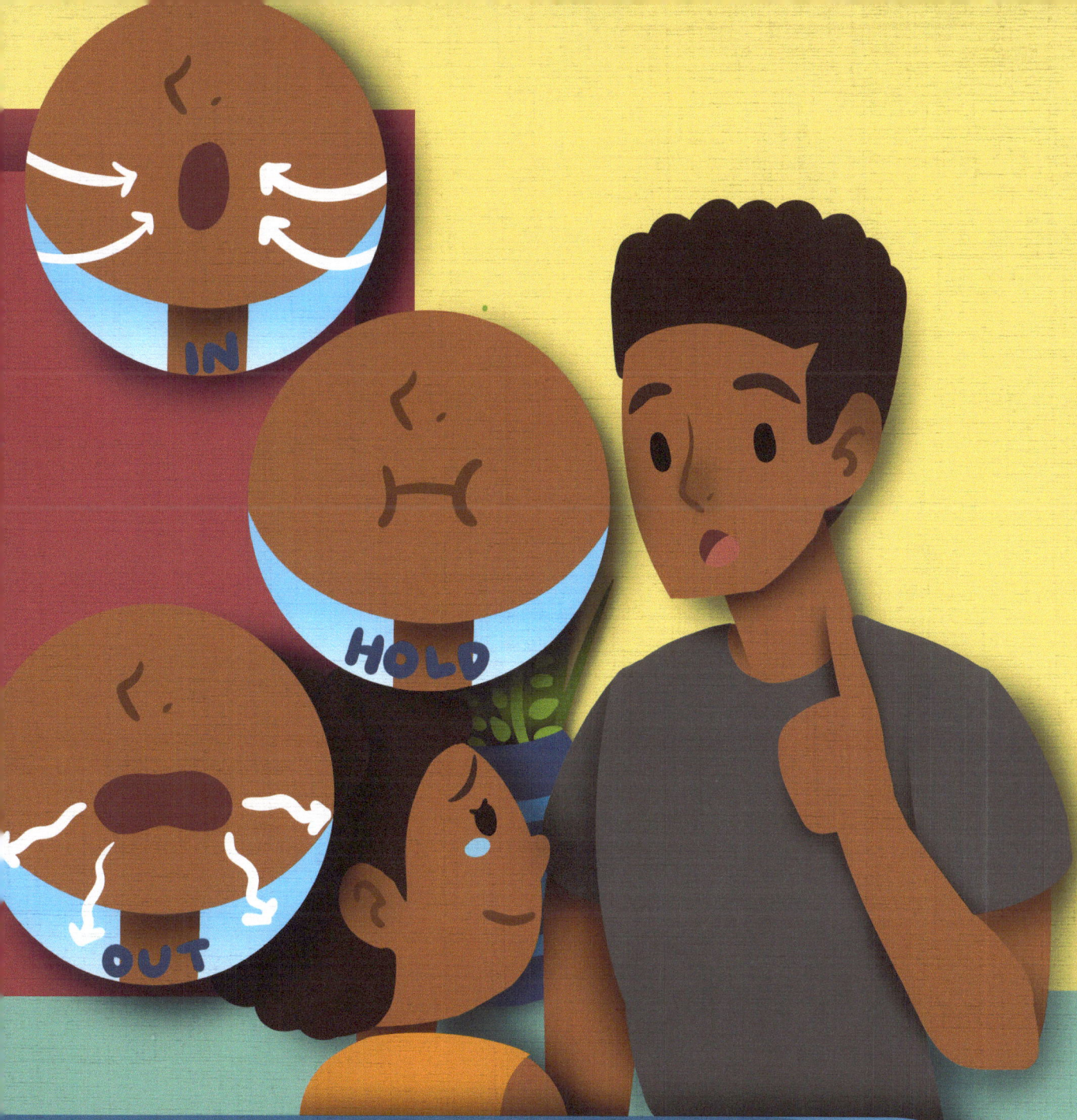

IN

HOLD

OUT

"Let's count and do it all together," said Dad.

"Take a deep breath for 1–2–3–4.
Hold for 1–2–3–4–5–6–7
and let it out for 1–2–3–4–5–6–7–8!" Dad counted, trying his
best to blow out slowly.

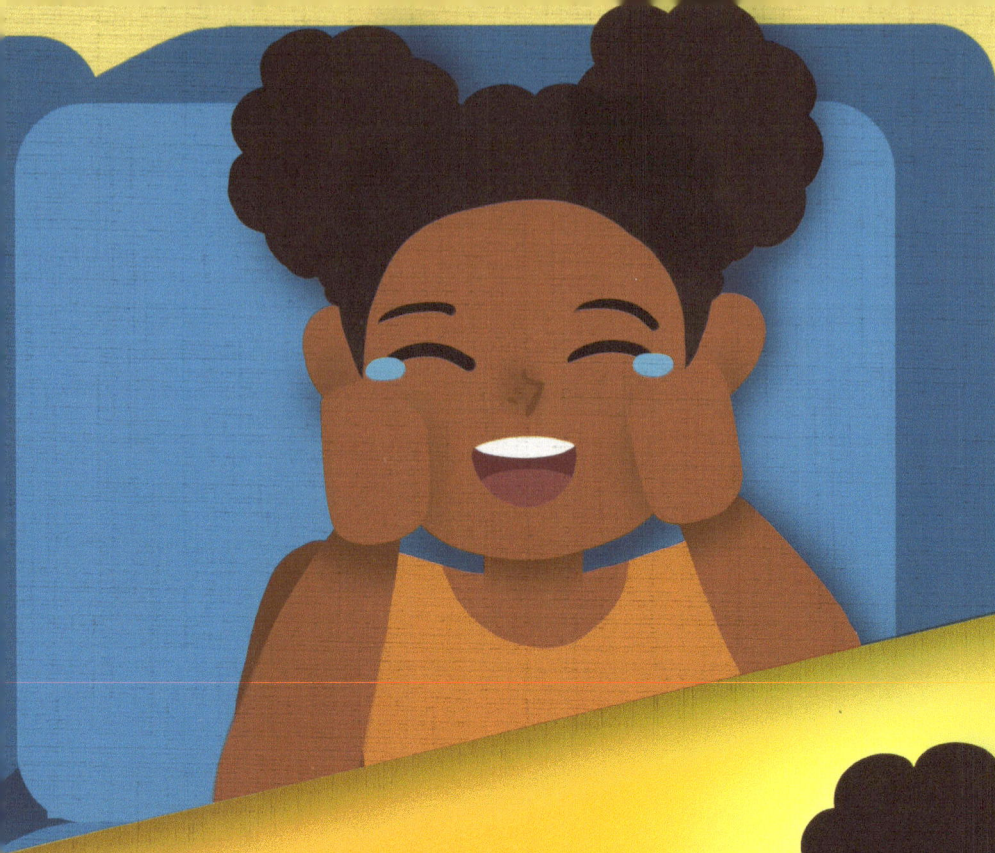

Samia's breathing slowed down, and she wiped away her tears. Samia asked, "Mom, may I wear my new pink gymnastics outfit tomorrow?"

"Yes, Samia, you may."

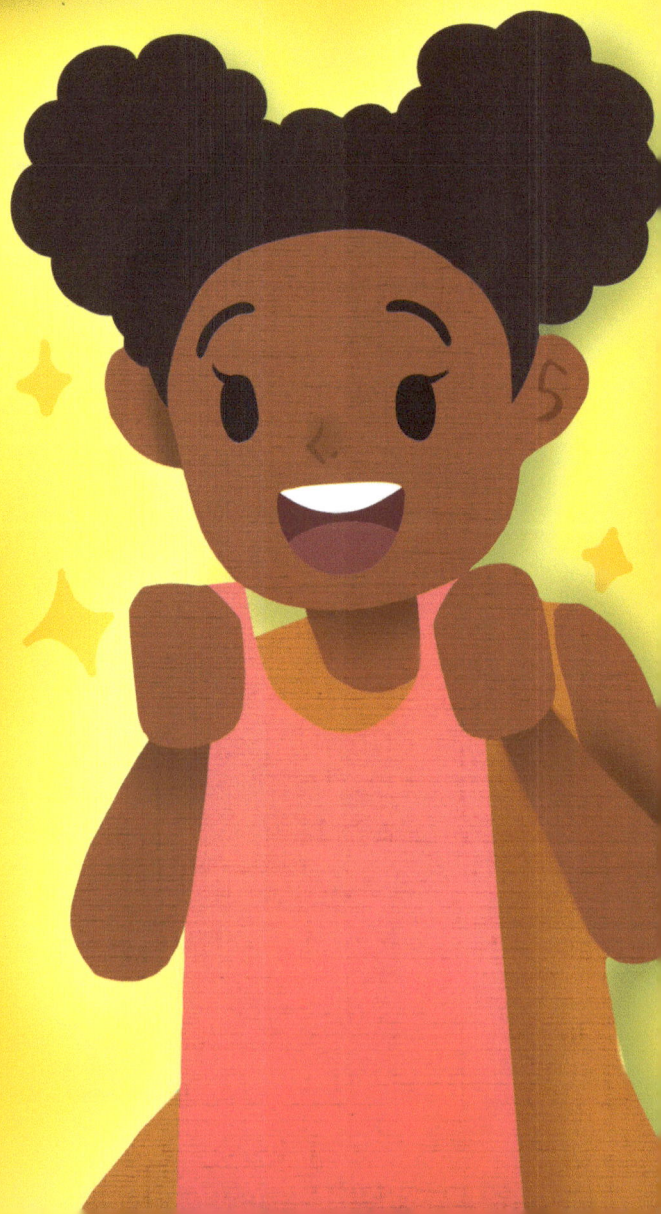

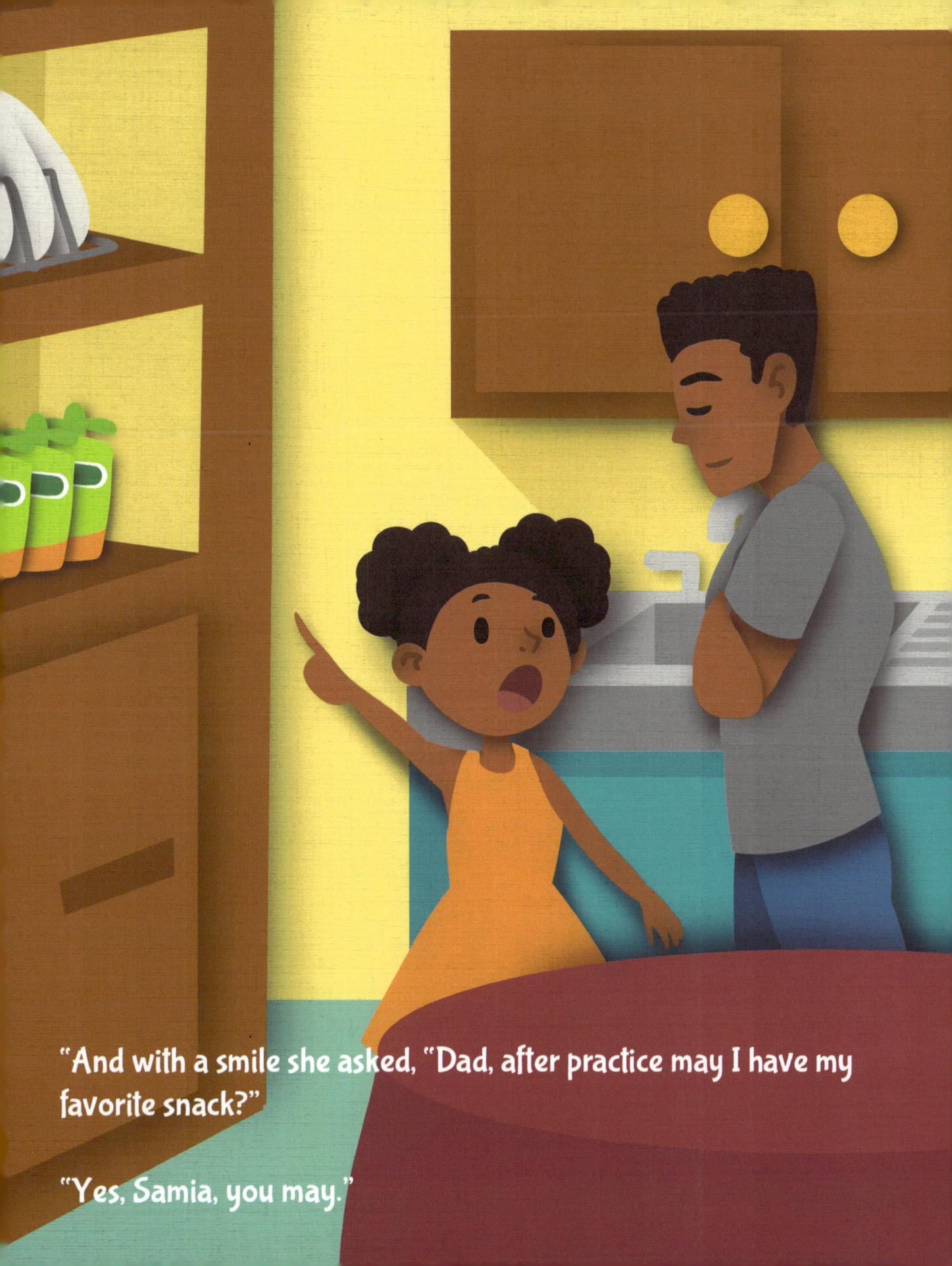

"And with a smile she asked, "Dad, after practice may I have my favorite snack?"

"Yes, Samia, you may."

"I'm so excited!" exclaimed Samia, jumping up and down. Samia went straight to her backpack to make sure she packed her outfit for the next day.

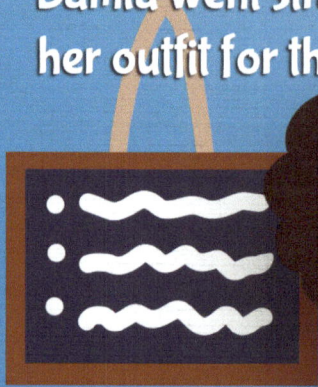

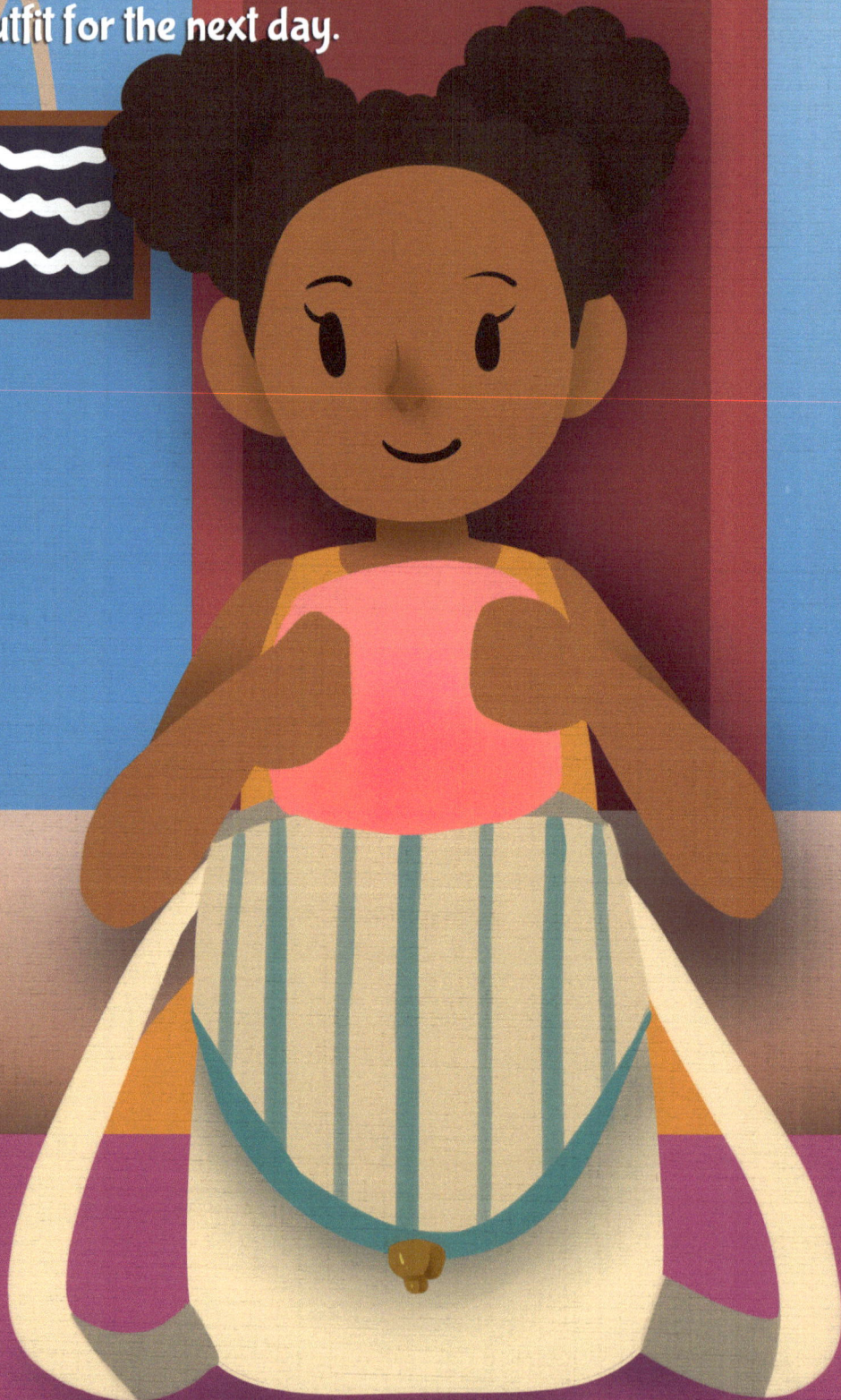

Samia went to sleep smiling.

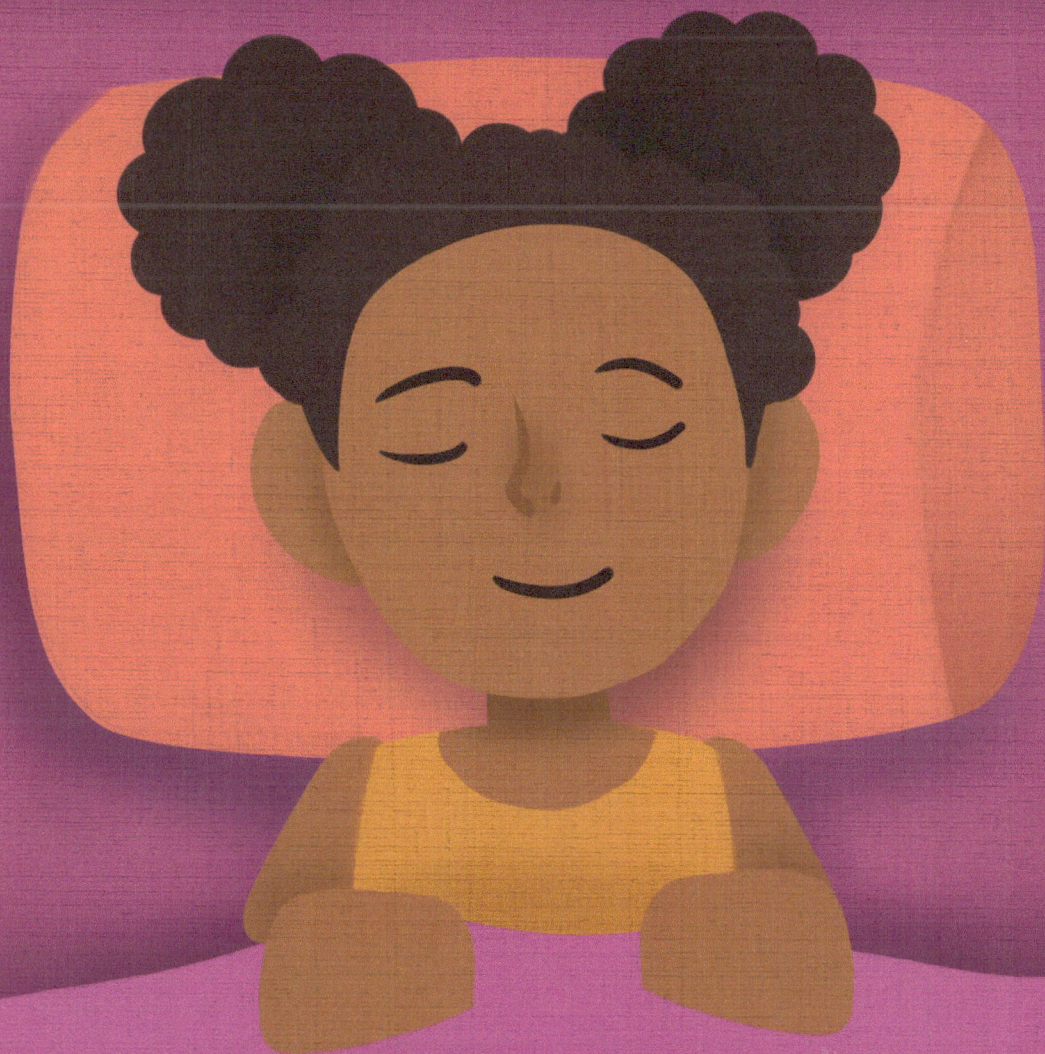

The next day, when Samia woke up early, she started to have doubts. "What if I forget my name? Or...or...what if I trip and fall?"

Her breathing got faster and she started to whimper again.

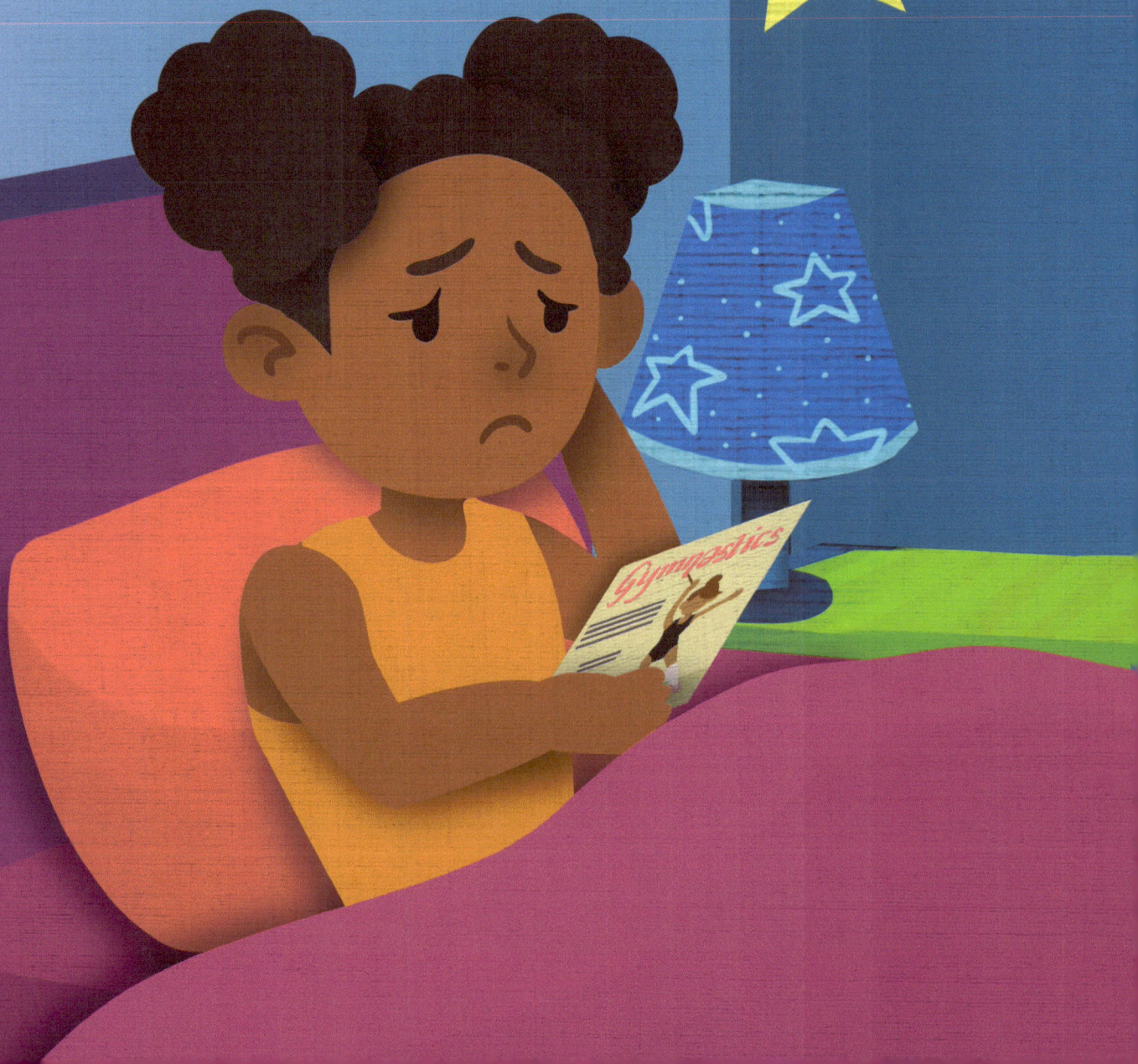

Then she remembered:
"Deep breath for 1–2–3–4.
Hold for 1–2–3–4–5–6–7
and breathe out for 1–2–3–4–5–6–7–8!"

She jumped out of bed. She got excited once again! Samia was ready for the first day of gymnastics class!

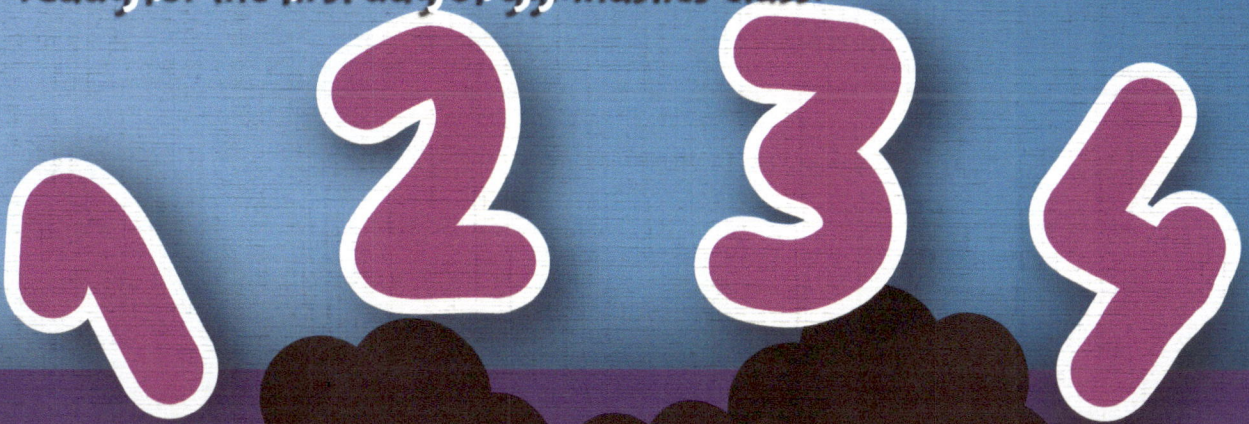

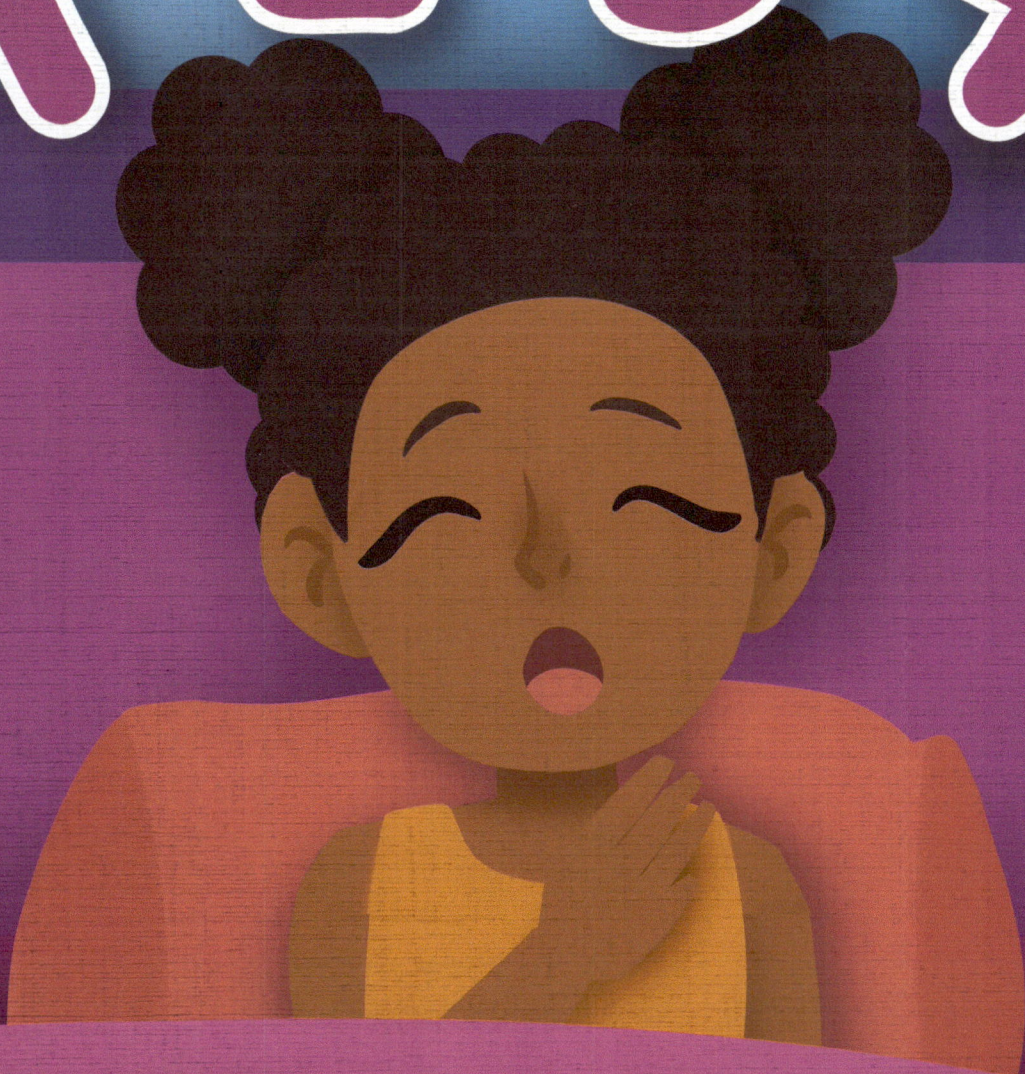

GYMNASIUM

Mom and Dad walked Samia to the gymnasium for her first day. Samia was smiling from ear to ear knowing that everything was going to be A—Okay!

When she got to the gymnasium, coach Sasha was there to greet her with open arms. Samia gave a big hug goodbye to her mom and dad. She took a deep breath and skipped her way over to join the rest of the class.

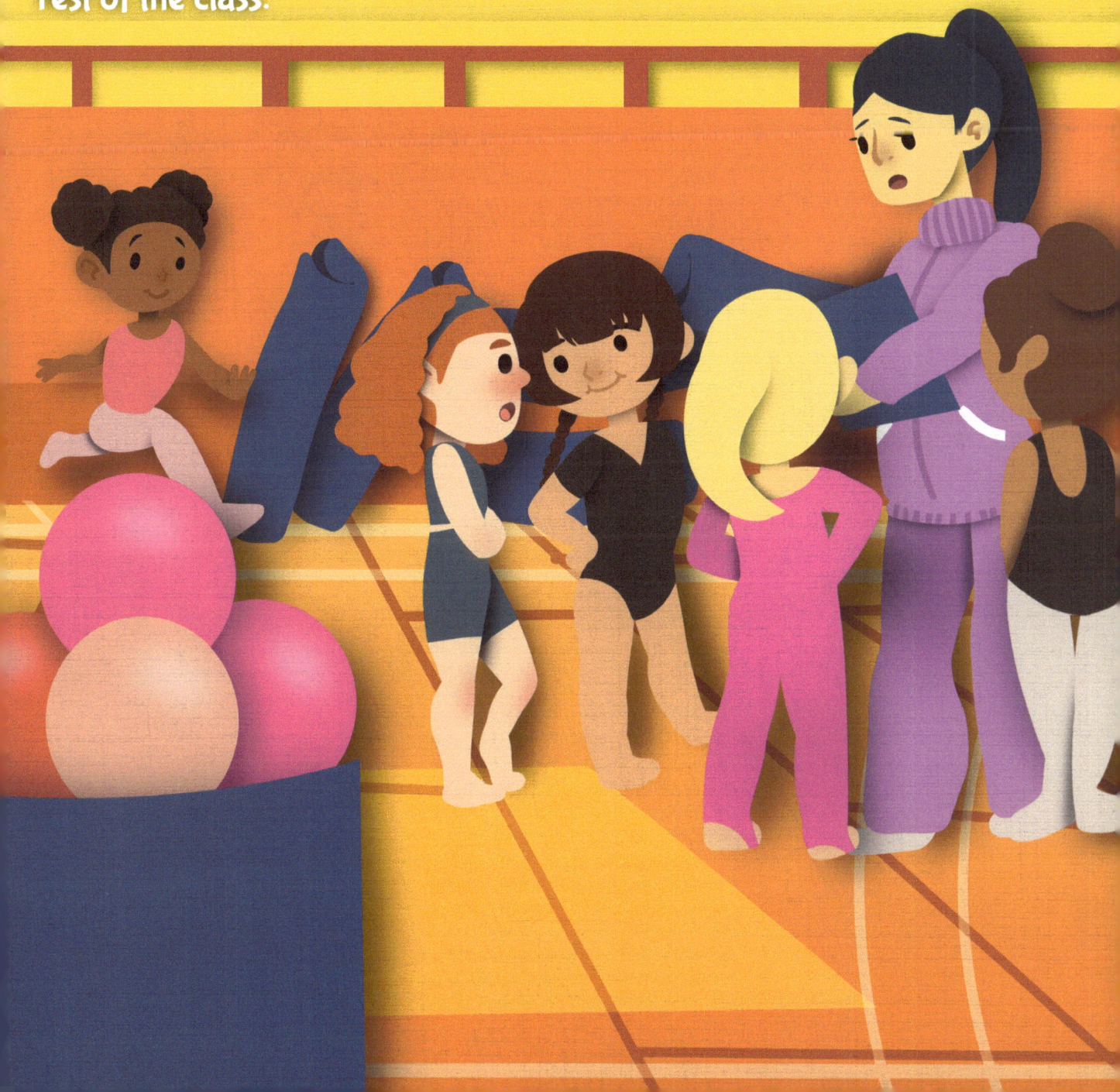

She was standing beside another new girl who was all by herself.

"Hello, my name is Samia. What's your name?" Samia asked.

The little girl said, "I'm...I'm...my name is...uh, uhhh."

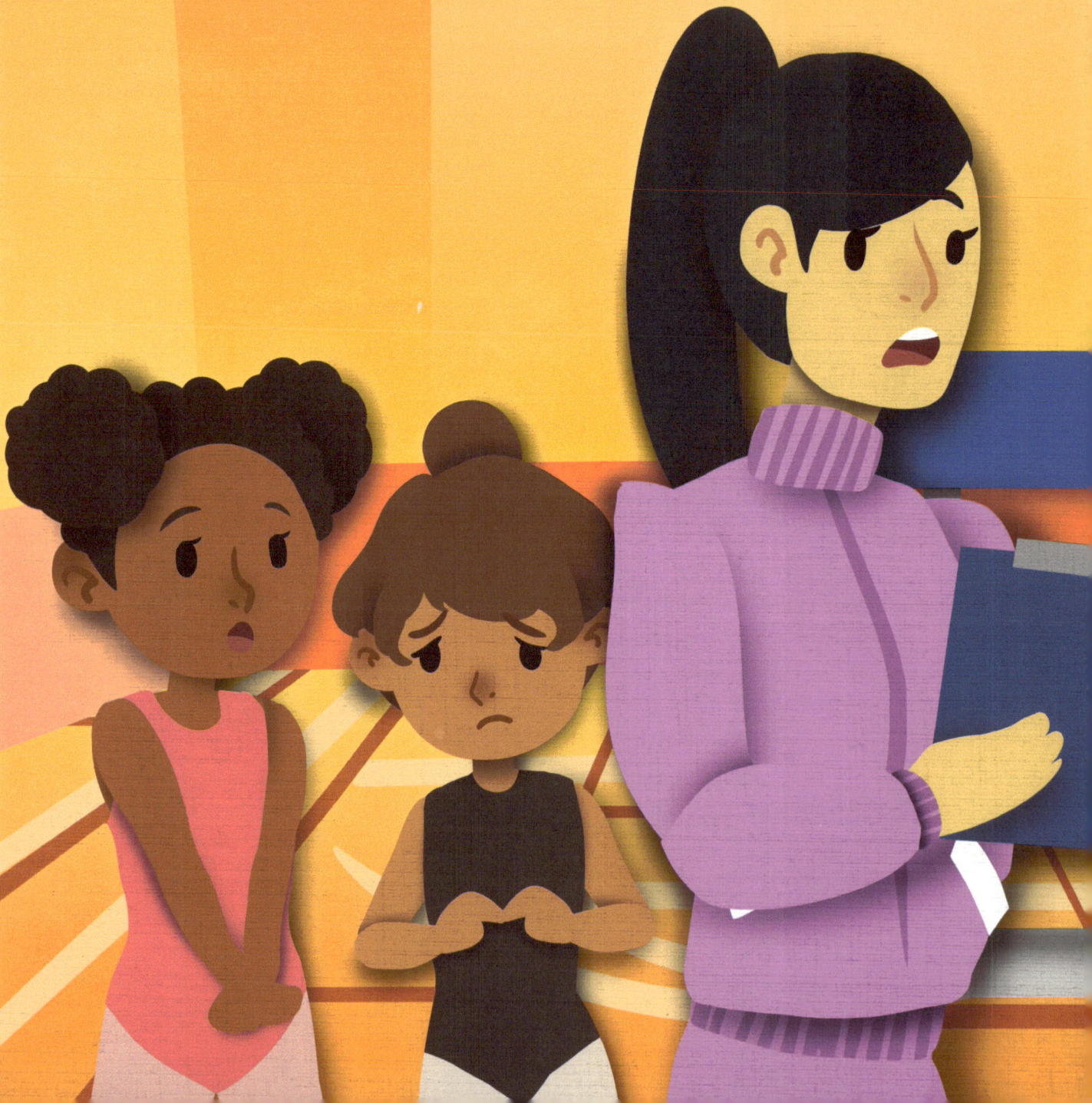

The girl started to breathe fast, her eyes welled with tears, her lips quivered, and she started to whimper.

"It's okay," said Samia, comforting the little girl. "I know a trick. Just do this and you'll feel a lot better!"

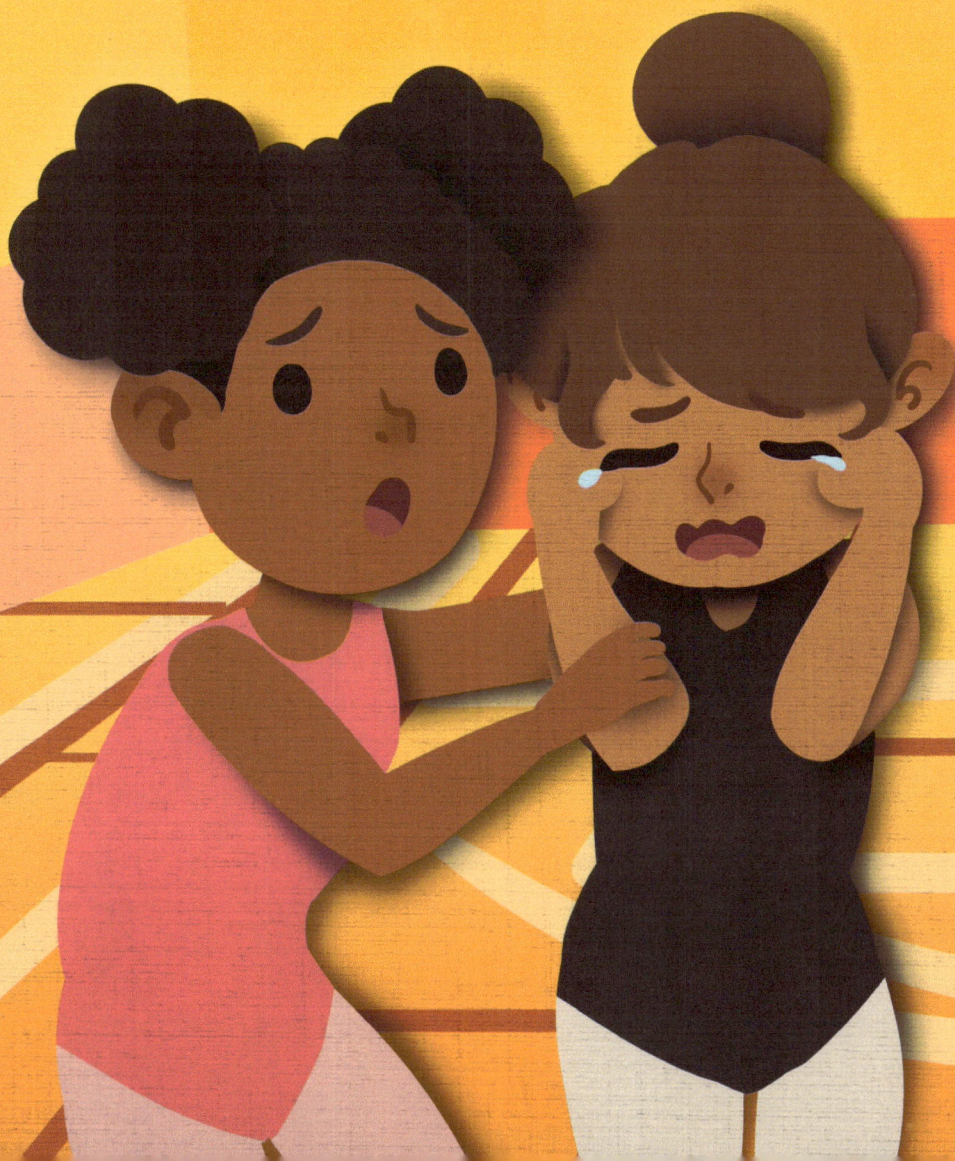

Samia showed her how to take deep breaths:
"Breathe in for 1–2–3–4.
Hold for 1–2–3–4–5–6–7
and out for 1–2–3–4–5–6–7–8!"

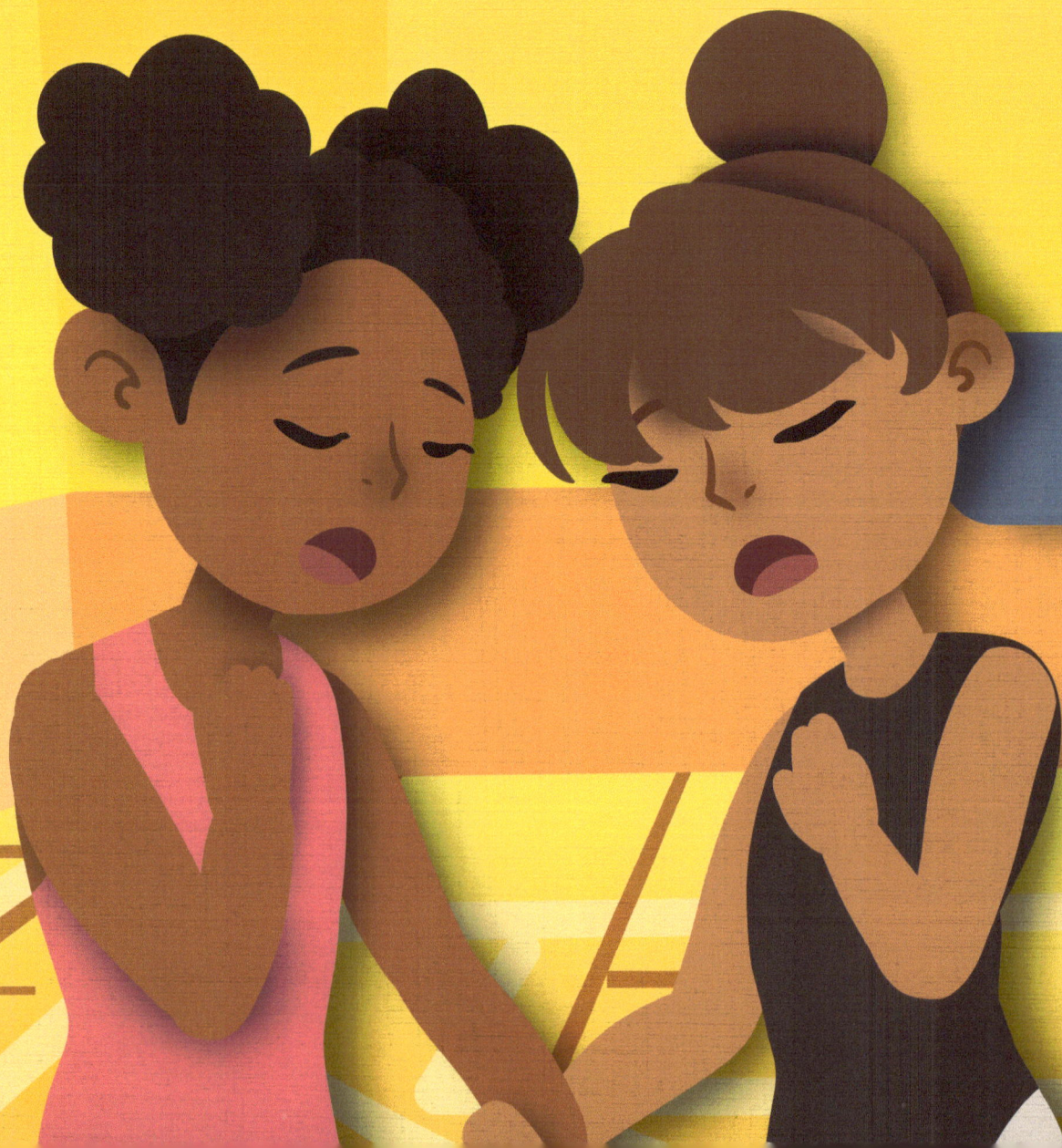

The little girl smiled and felt much, much better.

"My name is Melly," she finally said, and they quickly became friends. Together they hopped, skipped, jumped and flipped!

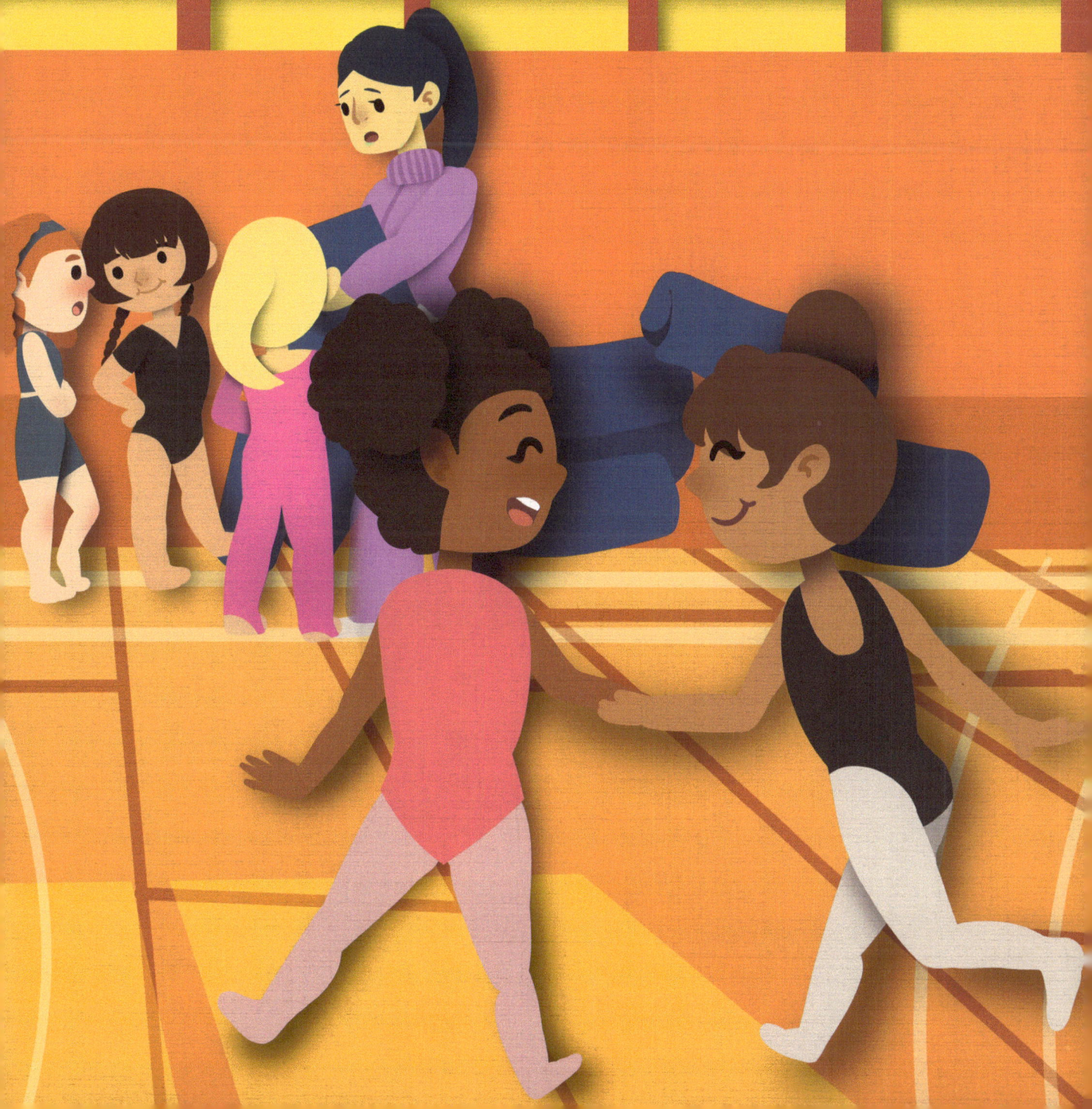

Samia had an amazing first day at gymnastics class.

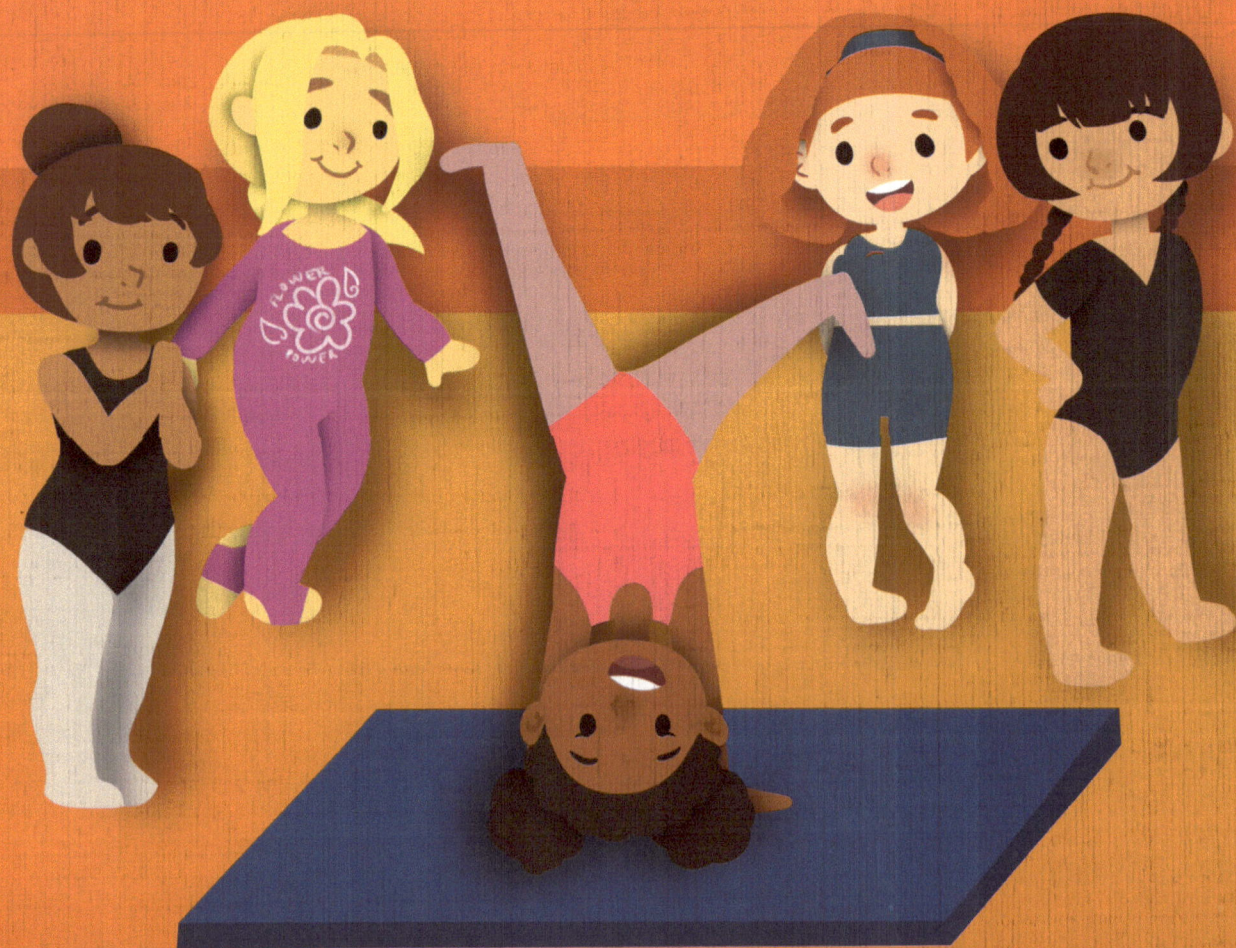

The End.

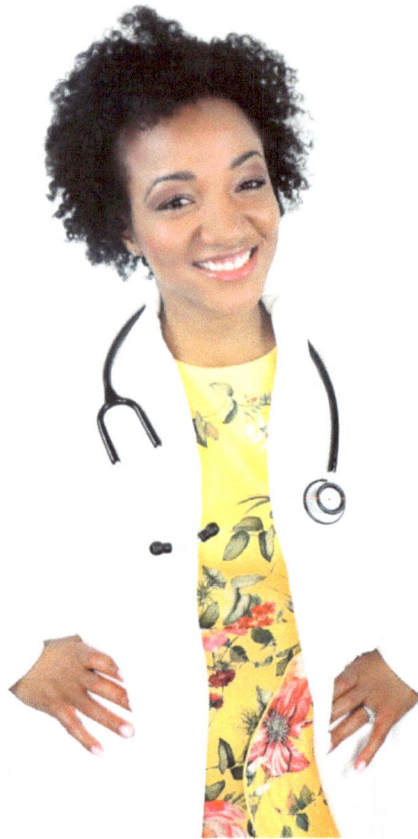

Dr. Cymanthia Connell is a board-certified family doctor born and raised in Montreal, Canada. She is affectionately referred to as "Doctor Cyam" by her family and "Auntie Cyam" by the younger ones including Samia. Dr. Cyam is a proud ambassador for healthy everyday living to prevent illness. She is currently practicing in the Greater Atlanta Area in Georgia.

Stay up to date with Dr. Cyam by visiting www.drcyam.com

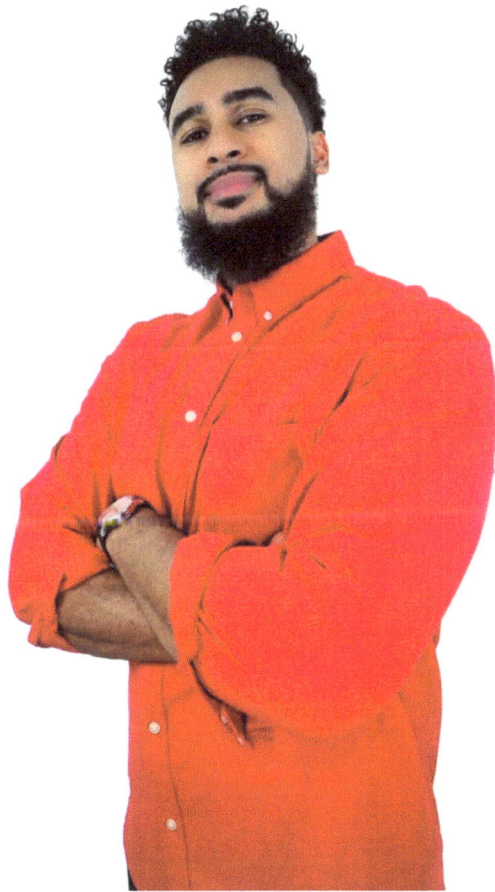

Adam Ali is a full-time online video creator based in Toronto and Atlanta with a passion for telling visual stories. He's excited to incorporate practical life lessons through his daughter's book series. After seeing his daughter's love for reading time, Adam became inspired to write a book with his daughter as the main character. He believes kids at this tender age can absorb some of the best lessons to shape their lives positively. He continues to inspire Samia to provide educational and fun messaging in her online videos and aims to do the same in future books too.

Stay up to date with Adam and Samia Ali on their family Youtube channel:
Youtube.com/TheAlis